Your Body,

Your Choices

A Woman's Guide to Reproductive Health and Birth Control

by
Mavis Korsah

MK Publishing

© 2025

Mavis Korsah

Copyright © 2025 by **Mavis Korsah**
All rights reserved.

No part of this book may be reproduced, stored in a retrieval system, or transmitted in any form or by any means electronic, mechanical, photocopying, recording, or otherwise without the prior written permission of the publisher, except in the case of brief quotations used in critical articles or reviews.

This book is intended for informational purposes only and does not replace medical advice. Readers are encouraged to consult a qualified healthcare provider regarding specific concerns or conditions.

First Edition
ISBN: 978-1-0682939-0-0
Cover design by MK Publishing

Printed and distributed by:
Amazon KDP and IngramSpark

Website: https://sites.google.com/view/mkpublishinguk/home

Dedication

To every woman who has ever felt confused about her body, misunderstood in a consultation room, or unsure of her options this book is for you.

And to the many young girls growing into womanhood,
may knowledge be your power, not your burden.

Mavis Korsah

Acknowledgements

I would like to express my heartfelt gratitude to all the women I have worked with throughout my career in Ghana and the United Kingdom. Your stories, questions, and strength inspired this book.

Special thanks to my colleagues, mentors, and former students who shaped my journey as a midwife and educator.

To my family and loved ones, thank you for your support, patience, and encouragement during the writing of this book.

Finally, thank you to every reader for choosing to learn, grow, and take ownership of your reproductive health. This book was written with you in mind.

Disclaimer / Author's Note

This book is intended for general education and empowerment. It is not a substitute for professional medical advice, diagnosis, or treatment.

Every woman's body is unique, and health decisions should be made in consultation with a qualified healthcare provider.

While every effort has been made to ensure medical accuracy, the information in this book reflects current guidance at the time of writing and may evolve over time.

Table of content

Chapter 1: Introduction to the Female Reproductive System 7

Chapter 2: The Menstrual Cycle 11

Chapter 3: Contraceptive Methods 16

Chapter 4: Natural Family Planning and Fertility Awareness............21

Chapter 5: Common Reproductive Health Issues 29

Chapter 6: Pregnancy and Fertility 35

Chapter 7: Postpartum Care and Family Planning 40

Chapter 8: Menopause and Midlife Health.....................................45

Chapter 9: Creating a Personal Health Plan 51

Bibliography..56

Chapter 1: Introduction to the Female Reproductive System

The female reproductive system is a complex and beautifully designed structure that plays a vital role in fertility, menstruation, pregnancy, and childbirth. Understanding its function is the foundation for taking control of one's reproductive health and making informed decisions about contraception and overall well-being.

The system is composed of both **internal** and **external organs**, with each performing specific roles. These organs are regulated by intricate hormonal cycles that prepare the body for the possibility of pregnancy each month.

1.1 External Reproductive Organs

Collectively called the **vulva**, the external reproductive organs include:

- **Labia majora and labia minora**: Folds of skin that protect the inner parts of the vulva.
- **Clitoris**: A small, highly sensitive organ involved in sexual pleasure.
- **Urethral opening**: The external opening through which urine exits the body.

- **Vaginal opening**: The entry to the vaginal canal, which leads to the internal reproductive organs.

These external structures also provide protection from bacteria and other pathogens and play roles in sexual function and childbirth.

1.2 Internal Reproductive Organs

These organs are located inside the pelvic cavity and include:

- **Vagina**: A muscular canal that connects the external genitals to the cervix. It serves as the passageway for menstrual flow, sexual intercourse, and childbirth.
- **Uterus (womb)**: A pear-shaped organ where a fertilised egg implants and grows into a fetus. Its lining thickens and sheds each month during menstruation if no pregnancy occurs.
- **Cervix**: The lower part of the uterus that opens into the vagina. It allows passage of menstrual blood and, during childbirth, dilates to allow the baby to pass through.
- **Fallopian tubes**: Thin tubes that extend from the upper uterus toward the ovaries. Fertilisation usually occurs here.
- **Ovaries**: Two small glands that produce eggs (ova) and secrete the hormones oestrogen and progesterone.

Organ	Function
Ovaries	Release eggs (ovulation) and produce hormones
Fallopian tubes	Carry eggs toward the uterus; fertilisation often occurs here
Uterus	Where a fertilised egg implants and grows
Cervix	Connects uterus to vagina; dilates during childbirth
Vagina	Passageway for menstrual flow, sex, and childbirth

1.3 Hormonal Regulation

The female reproductive system is controlled by a delicate balance of hormones, primarily:

- **Follicle-stimulating hormone (FSH)** and **luteinising hormone (LH)** from the pituitary gland in the brain
- **Oestrogen** and **progesterone** from the ovaries

These hormones regulate ovulation, menstruation, and the thickening of the uterine lining. Hormonal imbalance can lead to irregular cycles, fertility issues, or symptoms such as heavy bleeding or acne.

1.4 Importance of Understanding Your Body

Many women are never taught the full picture of how their reproductive system works. By learning about your body, you become empowered to:

- Recognise what's normal from abnormal
- Understand signs of ovulation and fertility
- Communicate confidently with healthcare providers
- Choose the best contraception for your body and lifestyle

This book aims to clarify these topics and provide accurate, respectful, and clear information to support your health.

Chapter 2: The Menstrual Cycle

The menstrual cycle is a natural, recurrent process that prepares a woman's body for possible pregnancy. Understanding this cycle not only helps in tracking fertility but also in recognising signs of health or imbalance.

The cycle is usually around **28 days**, but anything between **21 and 35 days** is considered normal. It begins on the first day of menstruation and ends the day before the next period starts.

2.1 Phases of the Menstrual Cycle

The menstrual cycle is divided into **four main phases**, each with 1distinctive hormonal changes and physical effects:

1. Menstrual Phase (Days 1–5)

This phase marks the **begining of the cycle**. The uterus sheds its lining, which leaves the body through the vagina as menstrual blood. The menstrual flow usually lasts between **3 to 7 days**. Cramping, bloating, mood changes, and fatigue are common within this phase.

2. Follicular Phase (Days 1–13)

Commencingt on the same day as menstruation, this phase is driven by **follicle-stimulating hormone (FSH)**. FSH stimulates the ovaries to develop **follicles**, each containing an immature egg. One follicle becomes dominant and prepares to release an egg.

Throughout this phase, **oestrogen levels** rises, which causes the uterine lining (endometrium) to thicken in preparation for a potential pregnancy.

3. Ovulation (Around Day 14)

Triggered by a surge in **luteinising hormone (LH)**, ovulation occurs leading to the release of a matured egg from the ovary. This is the **most fertile window** of the cycle.

Some signs of ovulation include:

- Clear, stretchy vaginal mucus (like egg white)
- A slight rise in basal body temperature
- Mild pelvic pain (known as *mittelschmerz*)

The egg remains viable for about **12–24 hours**. If sperm is present during this time, fertilisation may occur. Note: a sperm can last up to 5 days in a woman's body.

4. Luteal Phase (Days 15–28)

After ovulation, the ruptured follicle forms the **corpus luteum**, which secretes **progesterone**. This hormone maintains the uterine lining for a potential pregnancy.

If the egg is not fertilised:

- The corpus luteum breaks down
- Progesterone and oestrogen levels fall
- The uterine lining sheds, beginning the next menstrual cycle

If the egg is fertilised and implantation occurs, hormone production continues to support pregnancy.

2.2 Hormones Involved in the Cycle

Hormone	Function
FSH	Stimulates follicle and egg development
LH	Triggers ovulation
Oestrogen	Thickens the uterine lining
Progesterone	Maintains uterine lining after ovulation

2.3 Why Tracking Your Cycle Matters

Understanding your cycle can help you:

- Identify **fertile days** for natural family planning
- Detect irregularities or hormonal imbalances
- Prepare for your period and manage symptoms
- Know when to seek medical advice

Apps, charts, or journals can help track your cycle effectively. If cycles become irregular or symptoms are severe, it's important to speak to a healthcare professional.

28-Day Menstrual Cycle Overview

Cycle Day	Phase	Hormones	Events
1 – 5	Menstrual	↓ Estrogen, ↓ Progesterone	Shedding of uterine lining (menstrual bleeding)
6 – 13	Follicular	↑ Estrogen, steady FSH	Follicle develops, endometrium rebuilds
Day 14	Ovulation	Peak LH, ↑ Estrogen	LH surge triggers ovulation (egg released from ovary)
15 – 28	Luteal	↑ Progesterone, moderate Estrogen	Corpus luteum forms, endometrium thickens; if no fertilization, hormones drop

Chapter 3: Contraceptive Methods

Contraception allows individuals and couples to prevent pregnancy safely and effectively. Choosing the right method depends on personal preferences, health status, lifestyle, and future reproductive plans.

Contraceptives are generally categorised into **temporary** (short-acting and long-acting) and **permanent** methods. They can also be **hormonal, non-hormonal,** or **barrier-based**.

3.1 Why Contraception Matters

Contraception helps women:

- Plan and space pregnancies
- Prevent unintended pregnancies
- Manage menstrual-related conditions
- Gain control over reproductive choices

In addition to preventing pregnancy, some methods also offer protection against **sexually transmitted infections (STIs)**, particularly barrier methods.

3.2 Categories of Contraceptive Methods

A. Barrier Methods

These prevent sperm from reaching the egg.

- **Male condoms**: Worn over the penis; also protect against STIs.
- **Female condoms**: Placed inside the vagina; STI protection.
- **Diaphragm/cervical cap**: Dome-shaped devices inserted to cover the cervix; used with spermicide.

✓ *Pros*: Immediate protection, no hormones.

✗ *Cons*: May reduce sensation, must be used correctly every time.

B. Hormonal Methods

These alter the body's hormonal cycle to prevent ovulation or thicken cervical mucus.

- **Combined oral contraceptives (the Pill)**: Taken daily; contain oestrogen and progestin.
- **Progestin-only pill (mini pill)**: Taken daily and suitable for breastfeeding women.
- **Contraceptive injectables**: e.g., Depo-Provera, lasts 8–12 weeks. Norigynon, lasts 28 days.
- **Contraceptive patch**: Worn on the skin and changed weekly.
- **Vaginal ring**: Inserted into the vagina; releases hormones.

✅ *Pros*: Highly effective, can regulate periods.

❌ *Cons*: Possible side effects (nausea, mood changes), no STI protection.

C. Long-Acting Reversible Contraceptives (LARC)

- **Intrauterine device (IUD)**: T-shaped device placed in the uterus.
    - *Copper IUD* (non-hormonal): Lasts up to 10 years.
    - *Hormonal IUD*: Releases progestin; lasts 3–5 years.
- **Contraceptive implant**: A small rod inserted under the skin of the arm; lasts 3 or 5years depending on the type.

✅ *Pros*: Extremely effective, low maintenance.

❌ *Cons*: Must be inserted/removed by a healthcare provider.

D. Emergency Contraception

Used after unprotected sex or contraceptive failure.

- **Emergency contraceptive pill** (e.g., levonorgestrel): Best within 72 hours.
- **Copper IUD**: Can be used up to 5 days after unprotected sex.

✓ *Pros*: Backup option.

✗ *Cons*: Not for regular use, reduced effectiveness over time.

E. Natural Methods

- **Fertility awareness methods (FAM)**: Tracking ovulation signs (temperature, mucus, and calendar).
- **Withdrawal method**: Partner withdraws before ejaculation.

✓ *Pros*: Hormone-free.

✗ *Cons*: Higher failure rates, requires discipline and knowledge.

F. Permanent Methods (Sterilisation)

- **Female sterilisation (tubal ligation)**: Fallopian tubes are tied, clipped, or sealed.
- **Male sterilisation (vasectomy)**: Vas deferens are cut or sealed.

✓ *Pros*: Permanent solution.

✗ *Cons*: Surgical, not easily reversible.

3.3 Choosing the Right Method

Consider:

- Health conditions (e.g., hypertension, diabetes)
- Desire for future children
- Comfort with daily vs. long-term methods
- STI risk
- Cultural or religious beliefs

Consulting a healthcare provider ensures a method suits your needs and lifestyle.

Chapter 4: Natural Family Planning and Fertility Awareness

Natural Family Planning (NFP) and Fertility Awareness Methods (FAM) are approaches to birth control based on understanding and tracking a woman's natural fertility signals. These methods empower women to recognise their fertile window and avoid or achieve pregnancy without the use of hormones, devices, or drugs.

4.1 What Is Natural Family Planning?

NFP involves monitoring physical signs of fertility throughout the menstrual cycle to determine:

- When you are most likely to conceive (fertile window)
- When you are unlikely to conceive (infertile window)

By avoiding unprotected sex during fertile days, couples can effectively prevent pregnancy. These methods can also be used by those trying to conceive.

4.2 Types of Fertility Awareness Methods

Each method requires daily observation and consistent tracking. Some women combine more than one for greater accuracy.

1. Calendar Method (Rhythm Method)

This involves tracking the length of your menstrual cycles over several months (6 months) to predict fertile days.

- Count from the first day of your period.
- Ovulation typically occurs around **day 14** in a 28-day cycle.
- Fertile window is usually **days 10–17** of the menstrual cycle.

✓ *Simple and low-cost.*
✗ *Less reliable if cycles are irregular.*

2. Cervical Mucus Method (Billings Method)

Observe changes in vaginal discharge:

- **Dry or sticky** mucus = infertile
- **Creamy or cloudy** = possibly fertile
- **Clear, stretchy (egg-white)** = peak fertility

✓ *Provides real-time feedback.*
✗ *Requires comfort with daily observation.*

3. Basal Body Temperature (BBT) Method

Measure and chart your temperature every morning before getting out of bed.

- A **slight rise (0.2–0.5°C)** signals ovulation has occurred.
- You are most fertile **two days before** the temperature rise.

✓ *Increases body awareness.*

✗ *Illness, stress, or poor sleep can affect accuracy.*

4. Symptothermal Method - Combines:

- **Calendar**
- **Cervical mucus**
- **BBT**

✓ *More accurate than using a single method alone.*

✗ *Requires training and consistent commitment.*

4.3 Effectiveness of Natural Methods

When used **perfectly**, FAMs can be **up to 98% effective**. However, with **typical use**, effectiveness drops to about **76–88%**.

Key to success:

- Daily tracking
- Education/training
- Avoiding sex or using a barrier method during fertile days

Apps, charts, and fertility monitors can help support accuracy.

4.4 Who Should Use Natural Methods?

NFP may be a good option for women who:

- Want a hormone-free method
- Have regular cycles
- Are willing to monitor and chart consistently
- Follow religious or cultural beliefs that encourage natural methods

4.5 Limitations and Considerations

- Not suitable for those with **very irregular cycles**
- No protection against **sexually transmitted infections (STIs)**
- Requires **cooperation from partner**
- Less effective with inconsistent use

4.6 Enhancing Success with Natural Methods

- Take a fertility awareness course or consult a trained instructor
- Use physical charts or mobile apps to track data
- Understand that stress, illness, or travel can affect fertility signsTable: Comparison of Contraceptive Methods

Method	Type	How It Works	How Often Used	STI Protection	Effectiveness (Typical Use)
Male condom	Barrier	Prevents sperm entering the vagina	Every intercourse	✅ Yes	~82%
Female condom	Barrier	Lines the vaginal canal to block sperm	Every intercourse	✅ Yes	~79%
Pill (combined)	Hormonal	Prevents ovulation	Daily	❌ No	~91%
Injection (Depo)	Hormonal	Suppresses ovulation	Every 8–12 weeks	❌ No	~94%

Method	Type	How It Works	How Often Used	STI Protection	Effectiveness (Typical Use)
Mini pill	Hormonal	Thickens mucus, thins lining	Daily	✘ No	~91%
Implant	Hormonal	Prevents ovulation, thickens mucus	Every 3 years	✘ No	>99%
Hormonal IUD	Hormonal	Thickens mucus, suppresses lining	Every 3–5 years	✘ No	>99%
Copper IUD	Non-hormonal	Toxic to sperm,	Up to 10 years	✘ No	>99%

		prevents fertilisation			
Emergency pill	Hormonal	Delays ovulation	Within 72 hours post	✘ No	~58–85% (time-dependent)
Natural (FAM)	Natural	Track fertile window and avoid intercourse	Daily tracking	✘ No	~76–88%
Sterilisation (female)	Permanent	Tubes tied or sealed	Once only	✘ No	>99%
Vasectomy (male)	Permanent	Vas deferens cut/sealed	Once only	✘ No	>99%

By understanding your cycle and learning to observe your body's natural signs, you gain valuable insight into your health and fertility. Natural Family Planning is a powerful tool when used correctly, whether you're preventing pregnancy or planning for it.

Chapter 5: Common Reproductive Health Issues

A woman's reproductive system goes through many changes from puberty to menopause. During this time, several conditions may affect reproductive organs and hormonal balance. Understanding these common health issues helps women seek help early, prevent complications, and manage their reproductive health with confidence.

5.1 Menstrual Disorders

Menstrual health is a strong indicator of a woman's overall well-being. Some common issues include:

1. Amenorrhoea

The absence of menstruation.

- **Primary**: No period by age 15.
- **Secondary**: Periods stop for 3+ months after previously being regular.

Causes: Pregnancy, excessive exercise, eating disorders, PCOS, hormonal imbalances.

2. Dysmenorrhoea

Painful periods with cramps in the lower abdomen or back.

- **Primary**: Not linked to any medical condition.
- **Secondary**: Caused by an underlying issue (e.g., endometriosis or fibroids).

3. Menorrhagia

Heavy or prolonged menstrual bleeding.

Symptoms:

- Soaking through pads or tampons in under 2 hours
- Bleeding for more than 7 days
- Passing large blood clots

Can lead to anaemia if untreated.

4. Irregular Periods

Cycles shorter than 21 days or longer than 35 days. May be linked to stress, thyroid issues, or polycystic ovary syndrome (PCOS).

5.2 Polycystic Ovary Syndrome (PCOS)

A hormonal disorder causing enlarged ovaries with small cysts. Affects 1 in 10 women.

Symptoms:

- Irregular or absent periods
- Excess hair growth (hirsutism)
- Acne or oily skin
- Weight gain
- Difficulty getting pregnant

Management: Lifestyle changes, hormonal birth control, metformin.

5.3 Endometriosis

Tissue similar to the uterine lining grows outside the uterus — often on the ovaries, fallopian tubes, or bowel.

Symptoms:

- Severe period pain
- Pain during sex or bowel movements
- Infertility

Treatment: Pain relief, hormone therapy, surgery.

5.4 Uterine Fibroids

Non-cancerous growths in the uterus. Common in women aged 30–50.

Symptoms:

- Heavy bleeding
- Pelvic pressure
- Frequent urination
- Pain during sex

Management: Medication, surgery (myomectomy), or hysterectomy in severe cases.

5.5 Sexually Transmitted Infections (STIs)

STIs can seriously impact reproductive health if untreated.

Common STIs:

- Chlamydia
- Gonorrhoea
- HPV (Human Papillomavirus)
- Herpes
- HIV/AIDS
- Trichomoniasis

Symptoms: May include unusual discharge, sores, burning during urination, or none at all.

Prevention: Condoms, regular screening, and mutual monogamy.

5.6 Vaginal Infections

1. Bacterial Vaginosis (BV): Caused by an imbalance in vaginal bacteria.

2. Yeast Infections (Candidiasis): Overgrowth of fungus, often after antibiotics.

3. Trichomoniasis: A parasitic infection spread through sexual contact.

Symptoms: Itching, discharge, odour, irritation.

Treatment: Antifungal or antibiotic medication.

5.7 Cervical Cancer

Caused by certain strains of the **Human Papillomavirus (HPV)**.

Prevention:

- Regular Pap smears
- HPV vaccination
- Safe sex practices

Symptoms (in advanced stages): Irregular bleeding, pain during sex, abnormal discharge.

5.8 When to See a Healthcare Provider

Seek medical advice if you experience:

- Unusually heavy or painful periods
- Bleeding between periods or after sex
- Severe pelvic pain
- Foul-smelling or unusual vaginal discharge
- Changes in your menstrual cycle that persist

Early diagnosis and treatment can improve outcomes, preserve fertility, and enhance your quality of life. Listening to your body and seeking help when something feels off is a vital part of self-care and reproductive empowerment.

Chapter 6: Pregnancy and Fertility

Pregnancy is a natural but deeply personal experience that begins with the fertilization of an egg and results in the development of a baby in the womb. Understanding fertility, early pregnancy signs, and how to care for oneself during this period is essential to promoting a healthy pregnancy and safe delivery.

6.1 Understanding Fertility

Fertility refers to the ability to conceive and carry a pregnancy to term. A woman's fertility is highest during her **ovulation window**—usually around **day 14** of a 28-day cycle.

Key factors that affect fertility include:

- Age (fertility decreases after 35)
- Ovulation regularity
- Lifestyle (diet, exercise, smoking, alcohol use)
- Medical conditions (e.g., PCOS, thyroid disorders)
- Stress and emotional well-being

6.2 Signs of Ovulation and Fertility Awareness

Tracking fertility signs can increase the chances of conception. These include:

- Clear, stretchy cervical mucus (fertile cervical fluid)

- Slight rise in basal body temperature
- Mild pelvic pain (mittelschmerz)
- Increased libido

Apps, charts, and ovulation test kits can help predict the fertile window.

6.3 How Pregnancy Happens

Pregnancy begins when:

1. An egg is released from the ovary (ovulation)
2. It is fertilized by sperm (usually in the fallopian tube)
3. The fertilized egg travels to the uterus and implants in the uterine lining

6.4 Early Signs of Pregnancy

Some early symptoms may include:

- Missed period
- Tender or swollen breasts
- Nausea or morning sickness
- Fatigue
- Increased urination
- Food aversions or cravings

Home pregnancy tests detect the human chorionic gonadotropin hormone **HCG** and are most accurate after a missed period. A healthcare provider can confirm pregnancy with a blood test or ultrasound.

6.5 Prenatal Care

Prenatal care is essential to ensure the health of both mother and baby.

Key components:

- Early booking and regular antenatal visits
- Monitoring blood pressure, blood sugar, and weight
- Ultrasound scans to monitor baby's development
- Taking supplements (e.g., **folic acid**, **iron**, **calcium**)
- Screening for infections and complications

Pregnant women should eat a balanced diet, stay hydrated, avoid alcohol and smoking, and rest adequately.

6.6 Common Pregnancy Discomforts

While many symptoms are normal, they can cause discomfort:

- Morning sickness
- Back pain
- Heartburn

- Constipation
- Swollen feet or ankles

Gentle exercise, good nutrition, and supportive care can help manage these discomforts.

6.7 High-Risk Pregnancies

Some pregnancies require closer monitoring:

- Women with high blood pressure, diabetes, or previous complications
- Teenage mothers or women over age 35
- Multiple pregnancies (twins, triplets)

These women may need more frequent check-ups and possibly specialist care.

6.8 Preparing for Labour and Birth

As the due date approaches:

- Attend childbirth education classes
- Create a birth plan (preferred place of birth, pain relief options)
- Pack a hospital bag
- Know when to seek help (e.g., labour pains, water breaking, reduced baby movements)

Support from a midwife, partner, or doula can make the birth experience more positive and empowering.

6.9 Emotional Health during Pregnancy

Pregnancy can bring joy and excitement—but also anxiety or mood swings. Emotional changes are normal, but persistent sadness, fear, or disconnection may signal prenatal depression or anxiety. Talk to a healthcare provider if you feel overwhelmed.

Caring for your reproductive health includes preparing for pregnancy with knowledge, intention, and support.

Whether you're hoping to conceive now or in the future, understanding your fertility and pregnancy journey will help you make informed and confident choices.

Chapter 7: Postpartum Care and Family Planning

The postpartum period also known as the **fourth trimester** is the time following childbirth, when a woman's body, emotions, and lifestyle begin to adjust after pregnancy. Proper postpartum care is vital to physical recovery, mental wellness, and long-term reproductive health.

This chapter also explores how to make informed **family planning decisions** after delivery.

7.1 Understanding the Postpartum Period

The postpartum period typically refers to the **first six weeks** after birth, though full recovery can take months. During this time, the body undergoes significant changes as it returns to its pre-pregnancy state.

7.2 Physical Recovery after Birth

Key changes include:

- **Uterus involution**: The uterus shrinks back to normal size.
- **Vaginal discharge (lochia)**: Bleeding may continue for several weeks.

- **Breast changes**: Milk production begins 2–4 days after birth.
- **Perineal discomfort**: Pain or soreness after vaginal delivery.
- **Caesarean wound care** (if applicable)

It's important to:

- Rest as much as possible
- Maintain hygiene
- Eat nutritious meals
- Drink plenty of water

7.3 Emotional and Mental Health

Many new mothers experience:

- **Baby blues** (short-term mood swings, irritability, sadness)
- **Postpartum depression (PPD)**: Persistent sadness, hopelessness, disinterest in baby or life

If symptoms last more than two weeks, seek professional support. Emotional well-being is just as important as physical healing.

7.4 Sexual Health After Birth

It is safe to resume sexual activity when:

- Bleeding has stopped
- The body feels healed
- There is no pain or discomfort

Use **lubrication** if needed, especially if breastfeeding (which may reduce natural moisture). Communication with your partner is essential.

7.5 When to Seek Medical Help

Contact a healthcare provider if you notice:

- Heavy bleeding (soaking a pad in under an hour)
- Foul-smelling discharge
- Fever or chills
- Severe perineal or abdominal pain
- Signs of postpartum depression

7.6 Postpartum Contraception and Family Planning

Fertility can return **as early as 3 weeks** after birth — even before the first postpartum period. Choosing a reliable family planning method is important, especially if you're not ready for another pregnancy.

Lactational Amenorrhoea Method (LAM): If a mother breastfeeds exclusively and the baby is less than 6 months, fertility may be suppressed naturally. But this method is not 100% reliable and should be discussed with a healthcare provider.

Contraceptive options during the postpartum period:

Method	When It Can Be Started	Breastfeeding Safe?
Male/Female Condom	Anytime	✓ Yes
Progestin-only pill (mini-pill)	Immediately	✓ Yes
Contraceptive injection	Within 6 weeks	✓ Yes
IUD (copper or hormonal)	4–6 weeks postpartum	✓ Yes
Implant	Any time after delivery	✓ Yes
Combined pill	After 6 weeks (non-breastfeeding)	✗ No (if breastfeeding early postpartum)

7.7 Planning Future Pregnancies

WHO recommends spacing pregnancies at least **24 months apart** to reduce risks to both mother and baby. Consider your physical, emotional, and financial readiness before planning for more children.

Postpartum care is not just about physical healing, it's a time to adjust to a new role, care for your mental and emotional health, and make intentional decisions about your reproductive future.

Chapter 8: Menopause and Midlife Health

Menopause is a natural transition in a woman's life, marking the end of her reproductive years. While it is often surrounded by anxiety and misinformation, understanding menopause as a **normal and healthy phase** helps women navigate this period with confidence and self-awareness.

8.1 What Is Menopause?

Menopause is defined as the point when a woman has gone **12 consecutive months without a menstrual period**. It usually occurs between the ages of **45 and 55**, with the average age being **51**.

The transition happens gradually and includes:

- **Perimenopause**: The years leading up to menopause, when hormone levels begin to fluctuate and symptoms start.
- **Menopause**: When periods stop completely.
- **Postmenopause**: The years following menopause.

8.2 Common Symptoms of Menopause

Symptoms vary from woman to woman. Some experience very few, while others may need support managing them.

Physical symptoms:

- Hot flashes
- Night sweats
- Irregular periods
- Vaginal dryness
- Sleep disturbances
- Fatigue

Emotional symptoms:

- Mood swings
- Anxiety or depression
- Forgetfulness or difficulty concentrating
- Low libido

MENOPAUSE

Hot flashes

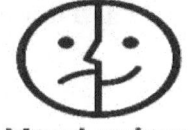
Mood swings

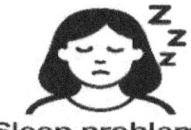
Sleep problems

Joint pain

These changes are primarily caused by a **decline in oestrogen and progesterone** levels.

8.3 Managing Menopausal Symptoms

There are both **medical** and **natural options** to manage symptoms:

Hormone Replacement Therapy (HRT)

- Replaces declining hormone levels
- Relieves hot flashes, vaginal dryness, and protects against bone loss

✓ *Highly effective*

✗ *May not be suitable for women with certain health conditions*

Non-Hormonal Treatments

- Antidepressants (for mood and hot flashes)
- Vaginal moisturisers or lubricants
- Herbal supplements (e.g., black cohosh, evening primrose — but consult your doctor)

Lifestyle Modifications

- Regular exercise
- Balanced diet rich in calcium and vitamin D
- Stress management (yoga, meditation)
- Wearing breathable fabrics to ease hot flashes

8.4 Bone Health and Osteoporosis

Postmenopausal women are at increased risk of **osteoporosis** due to reduced oestrogen. Bones may become brittle and fracture easily.

Prevention tips:

- Weight-bearing exercises (e.g., walking, light weights)
- Adequate calcium and vitamin D intake
- Avoiding smoking and excess alcohol

- Bone density screening as recommended

8.5 Cardiovascular Health in Midlife

Oestrogen has a protective effect on the heart. After menopause, the risk of heart disease increases.

Protective measures:

- Maintain a healthy weight
- Control blood pressure and cholesterol
- Exercise regularly
- Limit saturated fats and processed foods

8.6 Sexual Health and Intimacy

Vaginal dryness and low libido are common but manageable:

- Use lubricants or vaginal oestrogen creams
- Communicate openly with your partner
- Remember that intimacy and pleasure evolve — and that's normal

8.7 Mental and Emotional Wellness

Menopause is not just physical but an emotional transition, too.

Tips for emotional health:

- Prioritise sleep and self-care
- Stay socially connected
- Engage in hobbies and new learning
- Seek support if mood changes affect your daily life

Counselling or talking to other women going through similar changes can help reduce isolation or fear.

8.8 Embracing This New Season

Midlife is a time of great transformation — and great opportunity. Many women discover:

- A new sense of identity
- Renewed freedom
- Personal growth
- Time to pursue new passions or education

Understanding menopause as a **gateway** rather than an "ending" can be liberating. With the right knowledge and support, this chapter of life can be one of power, peace, and self-reclamation.

Chapter 9: Creating a Personal Health Plan

Knowledge is only powerful when it leads to action. This chapter helps you take what you've learned and apply it to your own life — whether you're managing your menstrual health, planning for a baby, preventing pregnancy, or navigating menopause.

A **Personal Reproductive Health Plan** is a tool to help you make informed, intentional decisions that support your body, your goals, and your well-being.

9.1 Know Your Body's Patterns

Start by tracking your cycle, symptoms, and health changes over time.

Track:

- Start and end of your menstrual cycle
- Flow intensity and symptoms (e.g., cramps, mood changes)
- Ovulation signs (e.g., cervical mucus, temperature)
- Unusual bleeding, discharge, or pain

Apps, calendars, or simple journals can help you build a clear picture of your body's rhythms.

9.2 Set Your Reproductive Health Goals

Ask yourself:

- Do I want to prevent pregnancy? If so, for how long?
- Am I planning to conceive soon or in the future?
- Do I want a hormone-free lifestyle?
- Do I need to manage specific conditions (e.g., PCOS, fibroids)?
- Am I approaching menopause?

Your answers will shape your choices.

9.3 Choose a Contraceptive (or Fertility) Plan

Based on your goals and medical needs, select a method that fits your lifestyle. Consult with a midwife, nurse, or doctor to find the safest and most effective option for you.

Include in your plan:

- Your chosen contraceptive method (or natural fertility tracking)
- When to start or review it
- Backup methods if needed
- Plans for switching or stopping

9.4 Regular Screenings and Check-ups

Make preventive care part of your health plan:

- **Pap smear**: Every 3 years (or as recommended)
- **HPV testing**: As advised
- **Breast exams**: Monthly self-exams and clinical exams
- **STI screening**: If sexually active with new or multiple partners
- **Bone density tests**: If over 50 or postmenopausal

Create a simple schedule in your journal, app, or planner.

9.5 Nutrition, Exercise, and Lifestyle

A healthy reproductive system depends on overall wellness.

Include in your plan:

- Balanced meals with iron, calcium, fibre, and healthy fats
- Daily hydration
- At least 30 minutes of physical activity most days
- Sleep and stress management techniques
- Avoidance of smoking, excessive alcohol, and harmful substances

9.6 Mental and Emotional Health

Reproductive health isn't just physical. Your emotional state influences hormones, libido, decision-making, and self-esteem.

Check in with yourself regularly:

- How do I feel emotionally?
- What support systems do I have?
- Do I need to speak to someone (counsellor, friend, faith leader)?

Include moments of rest, reflection, and self-care in your routine

9.7 Updating Your Plan Over Time

Your needs will change and that's natural. Revisit your plan:

- After childbirth
- If your cycle becomes irregular
- As you approach menopause
- When switching contraceptive methods
- After any major life or health change

Adapt and grow with your body.

Final Words

Taking ownership of your reproductive health is a lifelong journey and you don't have to walk it alone. With accurate knowledge, supportive care, and a thoughtful personal plan, you can live with confidence, protect your health, and honour your body through every season.

Your body is powerful.
Your choices are valid.
Your future is in your hands.

Bibliography

American College of Obstetricians and Gynecologists. (2020). *Your menstrual cycle*. https://www.acog.org/womens-health/faqs/your-menstrual-cycle

Centers for Disease Control and Prevention. (2022). *Sexually transmitted infections treatment guidelines*. https://www.cdc.gov/std/treatment-guidelines

Mayo Clinic. (2023). *Menstrual cycle: What's normal, what's not*. https://www.mayoclinic.org/diseases-conditions/menstrual-cycle

Mayo Clinic. (2023). *Polycystic ovary syndrome (PCOS)*. https://www.mayoclinic.org/diseases-conditions/pcos

Mayo Clinic. (2023). *Contraception: Birth control methods*. https://www.mayoclinic.org/tests-procedures/birth-control/about

National Health Service (NHS). (2023). *Periods*. https://www.nhs.uk/conditions/periods/

National Health Service (NHS). (2023). *Menopause*. https://www.nhs.uk/conditions/menopause/

National Health Service (NHS). (2022). *Contraception guide.* https://www.nhs.uk/conditions/contraception/

Planned Parenthood. (2023). *Understanding your menstrual cycle.* https://www.plannedparenthood.org/learn/health-and-wellness/menstrual-cycle

World Health Organization. (2021). *Family planning/Contraception methods.* https://www.who.int/news-room/fact-sheets/detail/family-planning-contraception

World Health Organization. (2023). *Menstrual health.* https://www.who.int/news-room/fact-sheets/detail/menstrual-health

Mavis Korsah

www.ingramcontent.com/pod-product-compliance
Lightning Source LLC
Chambersburg PA
CBHW060033040426
42333CB00042B/2432